baby massage

soothing strokes for healthy growth

suzanne p. reese

photographs by
bill milne

VIKING STUDIO

acknowledgments

Thank You

Vimala and the Circle of Trainers

Michael A. Curtis and Eric L. Babaian

Alice and Jose Gleria (aka Mom and Dad)

Doug, my beloved

VIKING STUDIO
Published by the Penguin Group
Penguin Group (USA) Inc., 375 Hudson Street,
   New York, New York 10014, U.S.A.
Penguin Group (Canada), 90 Eglinton Avenue East, Suite
   700, Toronto, Ontario, Canada M4P 2Y3
   (a division of Pearson Penguin Canada Inc.)
Penguin Books Ltd, 80 Strand, London WC2R 0RL, England
Penguin Ireland, 25 St. Stephen's Green, Dublin 2, Ireland
   (a division of Penguin Books Ltd)
Penguin Books Australia Ltd, 250 Camberwell Road,
   Camberwell, Victoria 3124, Australia
   (a division of Pearson Australia Group Pty Ltd)
Penguin Books India Pvt Ltd, 11 Community Centre,
   Panchsheel Park, New Delhi – 110 017, India
Penguin Group (NZ), Cnr Airborne and Rosedale Roads,
   Albany, Auckland 1310, New Zealand
   (a division of Pearson New Zealand Ltd)
Penguin Books (South Africa) (Pty) Ltd, 24 Sturdee
   Avenue, Rosebank, Johannesburg 2196, South Africa

Penguin Books Ltd, Registered Offices:
80 Strand, London WC2R 0RL, England

First published in 2006 by Viking Studio,
a member of Penguin Group (USA) Inc.

1 2 3 4 5 6 7 8 9 10

Massaging babies is a delightful activity, but as with any physical activity, please use common sense. Consult a physician before beginning. If your baby is crying or sleeping, wait until a happier moment. If your baby has a fever, diarrhea, has been vomiting, or appears in any way unwell, consult a physician. Neither the publisher nor the author is engaged in rendering professional advice or services to the individual reader. The ideas, procedures, and suggestions contained in this book are not intended as a substitute for consulting with your physician. All matters regarding your health require medical supervision. Neither the author nor the publisher shall be liable or responsible for any loss or damage allegedly arising from any information or suggestion in this book.

ISBN 0-670-03750-8

Printed in China

Set in Coquette and Adobe Garamond
Designed by Sue Livingston
Edited by Elaine Schiebel

contents

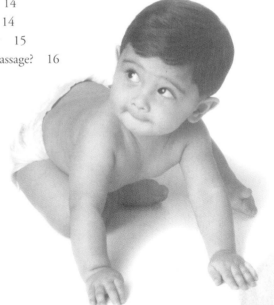

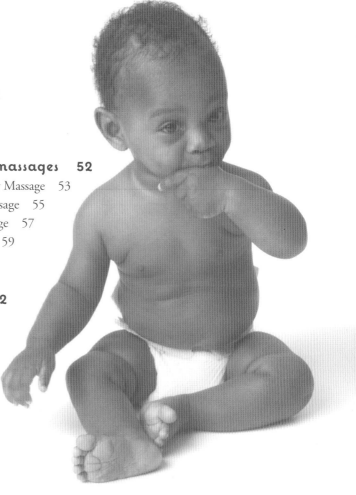

foreword

Mothers and fathers have been stroking and caressing their babies since the dawn of human existence, but in the helter-skelter world we live in now it's often difficult to find time to slow down to the pace that small babies need.

All lasting relationships are the result of many hours of meaningful interaction to find out what makes the other person tick, to uncover their personality, and eventually to discover the delight of simply being together. Babies need this time even more than adults do because their minds are only just developing, so it takes them longer to form these vital early relationships.

Small babies are particularly attracted to the person who brings them joy (when they're up for it) and who understands their needs when they cry. Baby massage is a brilliant opportunity for parents and babies to share time together and gain a stronger appreciation of each other. Initial guidance in baby massage techniques from a qualified and experienced instructor is a great help; even the most experienced parent can be helped to tune in to the baby's rhythms and to see how the baby is trying to communicate.

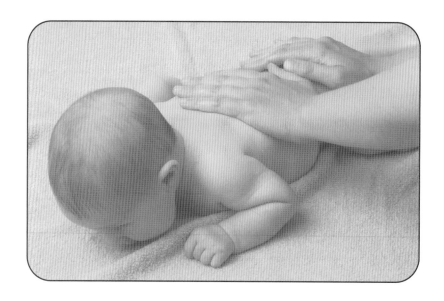

Baby Massage: Soothing Strokes for Healthy Growth focuses on giving babies the experiences that are most valuable for their physical, social, and emotional development, contributing to the lasting gift of high self-esteem. This delightful book is based on our current understanding of healthy child development and carefully avoids the half-baked theories of the past that have so often dismissed babies' need to feel felt, valued, and understood.

Sir Richard Bowlby, scientific photographer and son of the late Dr. John Bowlby, the twentieth century's preeminent expert on infant attachment

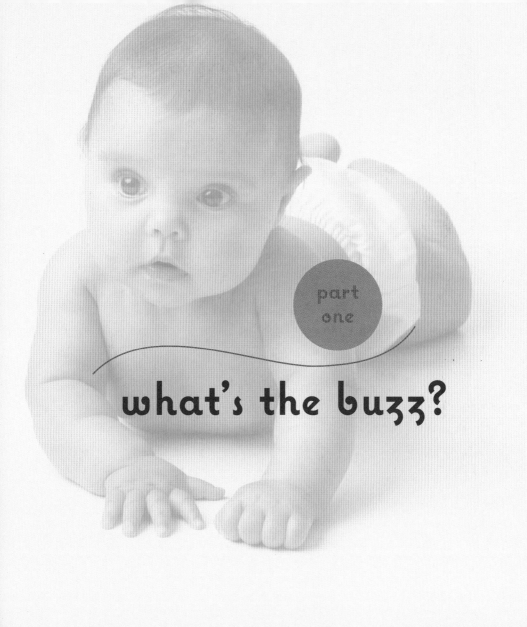

what's the buzz?

the buzz on the benefits of baby massage

What's the baby buzz about town and around the globe? Baby massage! Parents and babies alike are having a good time while also providing amazing physical, intellectual, and emotional benefits. But you don't have to take my word for it. Here is a sample of the buzz from experts around the world. (If you'd like to read the studies from which these conclusions have been drawn, see Buzz Sources on page 68 for the full references.)

* **Babies who are massaged before bedtime sleep deeper and longer and experience improved sleep/wake cycles—and that means you do, too!**[1]
* **Massage enhances infant learning.**[2]
* **Massage enhances immune function.**[3]

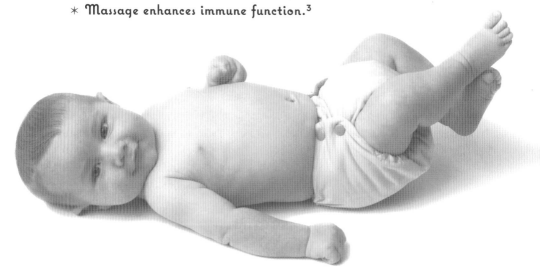

* Moms who suffer from postpartum depression become less depressed and feel less stressed when they massage their babies; they also experience more positive interactions with their babies.[4]
* When depressed mothers massage their babies, the babies experience greater daily weight gain, more organized sleep/wake cycles, less fussiness, and improved sociability and the ability to be soothed. Both Mom and baby experience improved interaction behaviors and secrete less cortisol and more serotonin (which means lower levels of stress and depression).[5]
* Fathers who massage their babies daily report feeling more confident and competent as caregivers and nurturers. Positive father-infant interaction increases.[6]
* With massage, infants experience increased weight gain, improved motor performance, and improved ability to handle stress in different states.[7]
* Preterm infants thrive on touch and gain more weight following as few as five days of massage.[8]
* Massage helps babies cope with pain while also reducing the sensation of pain.[9]

Baby massage is one of the healthiest things you can do for the development of your little one's brain, body, and the heart that lies between. Your little prince or princess will be more likely to sleep deeper and longer, eat and digest better, and cry less. So what are you waiting for?

can i really massage my baby?

Yes! From the day she is born. Because touch is the earliest of our five senses to develop and our earliest form of communication, the physical contact you've experienced so far—even if your baby is only a day old—means that you and your baby are already becoming massage pros. Touching, caressing, cuddling—all of this loving contact is a form of massage.

You will see that all of the massage strokes in this book are intuitive, so be bold! As long as you and your baby are having fun, you are doing it right. You and your baby will discover what works best for each time and place. No matter what massages you do, every time you massage your baby, you are sharing extra special time, and the positive effects will last for years to come.

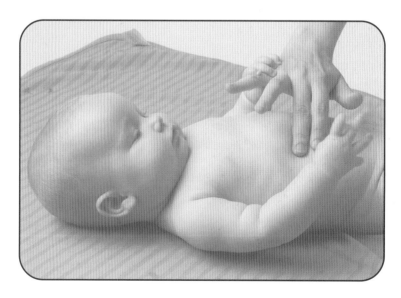

why massage my baby?

it's fun, it's easy, and it feels good

The key to the love connection between you and your baby is a hormone called *oxytocin*. Dubbed "the love hormone," oxytocin gives you that feeling you get when you hold your

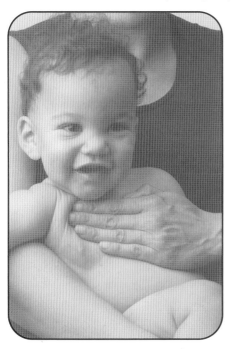

baby and never want to let go; it's the reason you feel better when you get a hug from someone who cares; and when it battles against the stress hormone cortisol, oxytocin wins! When you massage your baby, oxytocin is naturally released in both of you.

it deepens the love connection between you and your baby

Through massage, you and your baby are learning more about each other and the subtle cues and signals that you give each other. The trust and positive communication you are building will stay with you for years to come.

it can help your baby grow physically, intellectually, and emotionally

In addition to feeling great and bonding with your baby, science has proven that the simple acts of holding, hugging, rocking, and stroking your baby are helping your little one grow and thrive.

Your baby's brain is buzzing with new connections every day! By massaging a toe or a hand, you are introducing your baby to a whole new arena of body awareness and sensory discovery—really mind-blowing information for an infant! Studies have shown that this kind of early enriching relationship helps babies develop emotional good health and can even lead to your child's doing better in school and making friends more easily.

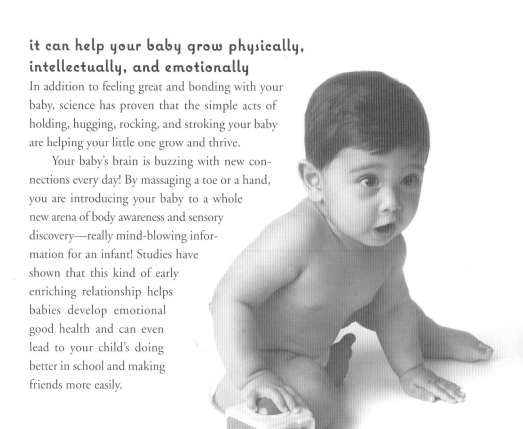

how do babies bond?

This chart shows how baby massage incorporates key elements of bonding. In general, bonding comes from shared experiences that help babies learn who you are, who they are, and about the love and connection you share. For infants, such shared experiences should always be positive, safe, predictable, and reliable. Baby massage incorporates all of these elements. This bonding can start at any time and will deepen with repetition.

eye-to-eye contact	Closely looking and gazing into one another's eyes; smiling and making funny faces at each other.
skin-to-skin contact	Hands-on, skin-to-skin contact, including touching, holding, hugging, rocking, stroking, and discovering that your baby has a strong grip.
sharing sounds	Talking, cooing, laughing, singing, and making silly sounds.
recognizing scents	You and your baby know each other by your natural essences. Without its being obvious, you and your baby recognize each other's scent signatures, and are comforted and reassured.

anytime?

Massage time can happen anytime, anywhere. While feeding, Mom can gently rub her baby's foot. While reading a story, Dad can rub his child's back. At bedtime, a brother or sister can rub the little one's hand. You can massage your baby sitting, standing, lying down, even with your baby on the move! Older babies may enjoy sitting in your lap, where they can see everything around them. All the massages described in this book can be adapted to a variety of positions that work best for you and your baby. Whatever and wherever is most comfortable for the two of you is what is right.

Nevertheless, there are times when your well-intended attention can become over-stimulating for a baby. During the massage, watch your baby for cues that say, "I need a break." As soon as you sense it, scoop up your baby for some quiet cuddle time.

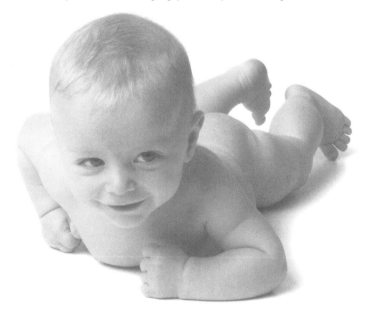

routine massage

Routine massage can lend itself to being a signal to your baby that something good and fun can happen . . . if she is up for it. Bath time can mean a fun, sing-along, bubbly massage. Soothing and relaxing strokes can help induce sleep. Stimulating and invigorating strokes can perk up baby when it's time to awaken. As part of your baby's day, massage will help him recognize his routine, and that can help everybody's day go much more smoothly.

social graces

Ask your baby, "Is this a good time for a massage?" Even though your baby cannot understand your words, he'll understand your intention and let you know whether or not he's in the mood. You know your baby best: look at his face and body and listen to his vocalizations. Your

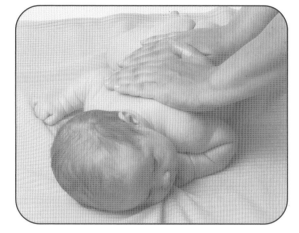

baby is telling you something. These nonverbal communications are really no different from the social signals we recognize daily: when to extend a hand for a handshake, how long to hold a hug, and how close to sit to people. Of course you want to show these same types of common courtesy to your very own bundle of joy! Don't forget—how your baby is treated determines how she will treat herself and others. Imagine a world in which everyone had been given massage as a baby!

how do i know if my baby likes the massage?

If you're not sure what your baby is trying to tell you, try the stroke three times, paying close attention to how your baby reacts. By the third stroke, you'll most likely know if your baby is enjoying it.

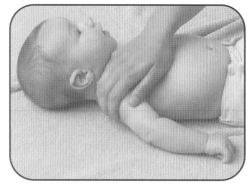

Look for more than one cue. He may be interested in something that's going on around him and be looking away, but if his body is relaxed and he's not crying, it's probably okay; trust your instincts on this—you'll know.

Try to keep your baby's interest throughout the massage. Talk to your baby about the strokes you are doing or sing a song—one of your baby's favorites or one that is recommended in this book. Throughout the massage, look for these signs that your baby is enjoying it:

* Your baby is making eye contact with you.
* Your baby has a relaxed expression or is smiling.
* Your baby's arms are wide open.
* Your baby's hands and feet are relaxed.
* Your baby is reaching for you.
* Your baby is holding your hand or arm while you massage.

anywhere?

Yes! There is so much flexibility in baby massage. Do it anywhere your baby is secure. If your baby is not at risk of rolling, falling, bouncing, or sliding out of your arms or reach, you're probably in a safe position.

You can massage your baby while sitting, standing, or lying down. Sit on a soft floor and keep him close, lying in front of you on a blanket. Try it while baby is lying on the changing table or sitting in your lap. If he wants to be held against you, in the over-the-shoulder burping position, for example, that's okay. Work with what he presents to you. As he grows, he might prefer to sit up in your lap where he can see his surroundings. Do it at home or away from home—whatever and wherever is comfortable for the two of you is what will work.

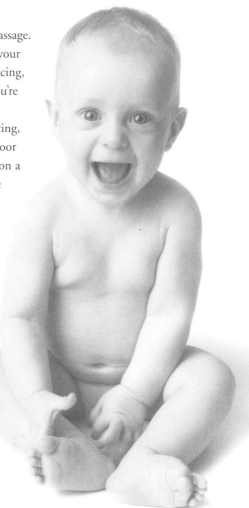

what body part do i start with?

The legs, feet, or back are usually good places to start, but really, you can start anywhere your baby lets you know it feels good. Once your baby gets used to the massage, the two of you will discover which parts are best to massage and when.

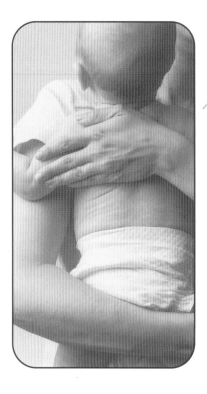

what kind of pressure do i use?

Be gentle yet firm. If the strokes are too light—featherlike—they could tickle, and that's a different experience! Feel your hands and fingers relax, mold to, and hold your baby's body. To start, place your hands on your baby's body—try the arm, shoulder, or thigh—and then mold and hold for a few seconds. This alone can be as powerful as a stroke and is a great way to introduce massage to a baby—especially one who's fussy at first.

When massaging, feel your fingers curl and curve around every roll. With gentle, firm strokes you are signaling to your baby that you are there, he is safe, and you love him.

how long do i massage my baby?

Because baby massage is not a spa session, the only way to know how long to massage is by paying attention to what your baby is telling you. As long as your baby's cues say yes and you are still comfortable, keep going. The massage can last just a few moments or it can extend to many minutes—there is no set length of time.

When you are done, be sure to tell your baby, "All done!" and finish off with one final sweep. Your baby will come to learn the cues that signal the beginning and end of the massage.

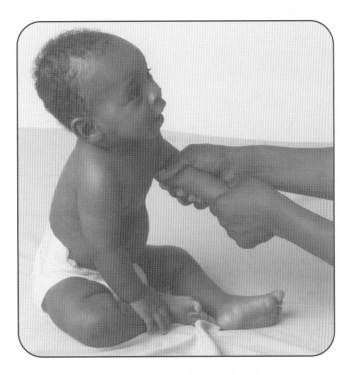

when are children
too old for massage?

Never! With massage as part of your family's life, loving touch can be a form of communication that bridges the all-too-familiar gap between parents and children.

toddlers	For these little bundles of energy, healthy touch can be combined with fun and games. "I'm gonna get you!" creates massage-on-the-move, and tots love the chase.
preschoolers and up	As your child grows, modesty will naturally increase and more clothing will remain on, but that doesn't mean massage has to stop. In fact, children at this "me-do-it" stage will often reciprocate with a well-deserved massage for you! Custom-tailor massages to what interests your child: create the Spiderman Special or the Ballerina Massage.
adolescents	The same kid who doesn't want you to kiss or hug her in public will still come to you when she needs your support. As you ease the symptoms of a sore shoulder or a headache, you are providing a safe space for what many parents call "the only time my kid really talks to me." Not only is a massage a wonderful—and perhaps rare—opportunity to share time with your adolescent, but he is learning positive and respectful ways to seek out and provide comfort as an adult.

what do i need?

As a loving parent, you have most of the equipment already! If you are in a place where it's not practical to remove any of your baby's clothing, then you can practice the strokes over her clothing. If you can take some clothes off, or even fold them out of the way to get some skin-to-skin contact, then use a bit of oil.

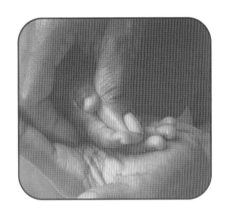

oil, not lotion

Because our little gnawers and chewers like to use body parts as their first lollipops, they will inevitably end up with oil in and around their mouths. So you need to make sure that whatever you put *on* your baby's body is something that you won't mind being *in* it. And like any food, it should be good and nourishing.

Look for unscented, unflavored, food-grade fruit or vegetable oil. Ask yourself: Would I cook or bake with this? Would I be comfortable feeding this oil to my baby? Is this oil food? If you can answer "yes" to all those questions, then you most likely have something that will work.

If you need to go out and buy oil, then go to the baking aisle of the market and look for plain and all-natural fruit or vegetable oils. Good choices are:

* grapeseed oil
* safflower oil
* apricot kernel oil
* olive oil
* almond oil (botanically, it is a fruit)

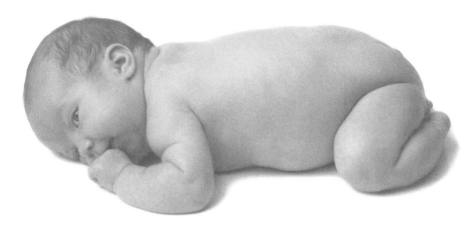

It's wise to do a patch test before rubbing anything all over your baby's body. Rub a dab of oil into your baby's skin on an area he can't easily scratch or rub, such as the upper back. Wait fifteen to thirty minutes. If no change of skin color or texture appears, then the oil is probably agreeable.

Which oils *do not* meet the criteria for food-grade fruit or vegetable oil?

* **Any commercial bath or beauty oil.** Even if it was made from a fruit or vegetable, would you eat it?
* **Any scented or flavored oil.** In addition to potentially being irritating to the skin or harmful if swallowed, scents and flavors can provide far too much stimulation for a baby and her developing internal systems. Also, your little one recognizes you and is comforted by your natural scent signature—why mess with that?
* **Baby oil or mineral oil.** Baby oil is mineral oil, often with a fragrance added, and should be avoided. It is a highly flammable derivative of petroleum, and if breathed in, it can lead to chemical pneumonia, irreversible lung damage, and even death.

a note on crying

Crying is an infant state like being asleep or awake—it's just what babies do. When babies express themselves vocally, it's often through crying. For this reason, crying should be celebrated. I realize that trying to remember that at three in the morning is tough. When your baby cries, it is because he needs you—you are his world, and you are the person he can count on to help him feel safe. If your baby starts to cry, it doesn't mean you're doing anything wrong; it means your baby is trying to tell you something: he may be tired, hungry, cold, or bored. He might just want to cuddle. You know your baby best. Talk to him, hold him, and let him know you are there for him. When you both are calm, you can proceed with a massage.

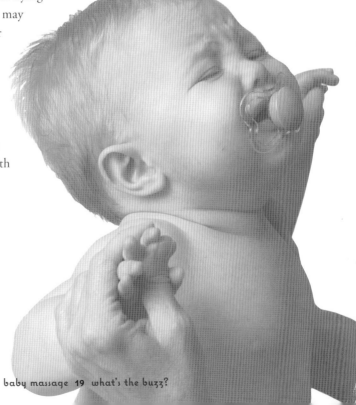

relax—first you, then baby

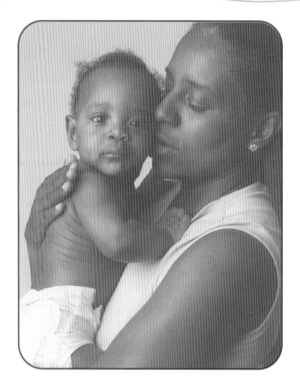

Your baby is a smart cookie. If you are preoccupied or in a sour or flat mood, your baby will know and, chances are, she won't be in the mood for a massage. Turn sour into sweet or just help sweet be sweeter! Before you begin, take a deep breath, roll your shoulders, and think of something relaxing, happy, or all-around good. Enjoy this *ahhhhhh* moment. Just by thinking warm and fuzzy thoughts, your oxytocin level is increasing. Now, it's time to share that feeling with your baby.

touching tips

Look for the boxes throughout parts two and three for more Touching Tips.

* Always watch your baby for cues, signs, and signals about how she is feeling.

* If your baby seems fussy or uncomfortable, yet seems to be physically fine, consider the environment. Are there bright lights overhead? Is it chilly in the room? Is the day hot or humid? Is there a strong smell? Check clothing or jewelry—is there something irritating your baby? A simple adjustment may be all that is needed.

* Massaging "up" your baby's arms and legs is invigorating. Massaging "down" your baby's arms and legs is more relaxing.

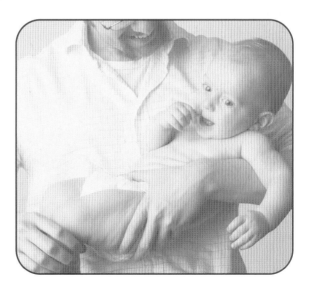

* Massage each part of the body as long as your baby and you are enjoying it, then try a new massage or part of the body—or take a break.

* Don't worry about getting the stroke perfect. You'll know what's working from the happy cues your baby is sending you.

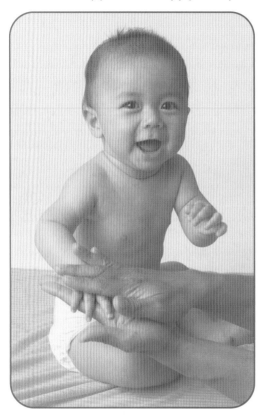

* Feel free to create your own adaptations, as long as the baby is safe and comfortable and you're both enjoying it.

* When the massage is over or when you are done with one part of the body and wish to move on to another, say to your baby, "All done!" and give one final sweep on that body part.

* Talk, tell stories, recite rhymes, sing, and dance!

* Have fun!

class

CLASS is an acronym to help you remember the starting sequence of any massage. Before every massage or when moving from one part of the body to another, make sure you do it with CLASS:

Contact: Make physical contact with your baby; rest your hands on the part of his body you want to massage. Relax, feel your hands mold over his body—mold and hold.

Look: Look at her, even if she's not looking at you. There is no need to force eye contact. What are her face and body saying?

Ask: Ask him out loud, in a soft whisper, "Is this a good time for a massage?" It's not the words that communicate. It's the intention behind the words that say, "I care about how you feel, and you are in control of your body."

Swish: Put a bit of oil in your hand and swish your hands together. Let your baby hear the swish of your hands. Even if you won't be using oil, swish anyway as your signal to her. Whenever you need more oil, add it and swish.

Show: Show your hands to your baby. Smile and hold your hands over her, so she can still see your face, and show her the tools you'll use.

The routine and rhythm of CLASS help your baby learn "it's massage time," and the anticipation of the massage can help him begin to relax.

for each massage

Each massage begins with "Relax and do CLASS" as the first step. This is a reminder to remain relaxed throughout the massage and make sure you go through all the steps of CLASS. If you are changing the stroke but remaining on the same part of her body, you only need CLA—Contact, Look at your baby's cues and signals, and Ask him if he is comfortable with the new stroke. Talking with your baby is so important. If your baby gives you the signals that he would like to be massaged, go for it!

Every massage ends with the same final step: when the massage is over, say, "All done!" and finish off with one final sweep. If your baby becomes fussy or it's just time to stop or move to another body part, say to your baby, "All done!" in that sing-song voice (known as "motherese") and do one final sweep of the body part. This signals to your baby that this is the end of a stroke or the massage. Congratulate yourselves with lots of hugs and kisses.

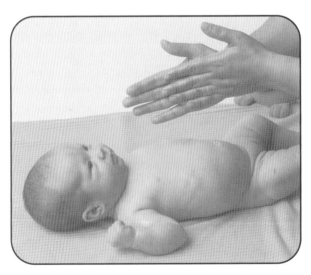

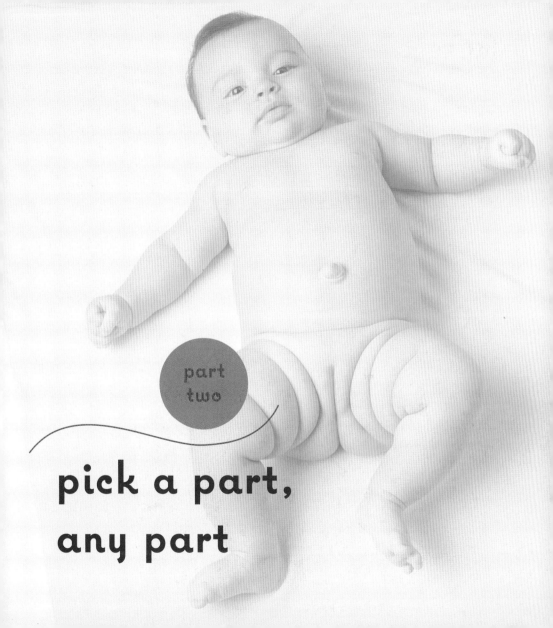

part
two

pick a part,
any part

legs

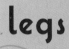

strokes: Slide & Glide, Swirl & Slide
song suggestion: "Wheels on the Bus"

The legs are often a good place to start
when introducing your baby to massage.
Most babies are receptive to having their
legs touched because the legs are far from
the face and are generally less sensitive.

slide & glide

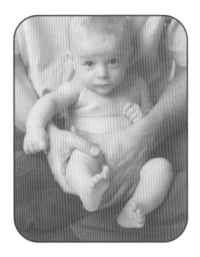

1   Relax and do CLASS.

2   Wrap your hands and fingers around her leg so your fingers make a C shape that molds to the shape of her leg. One hand starts high on the leg near her bottom. The other hand—in the same position—is just beneath the first hand placement.

3   Glide, using alternating hands, all the way to her ankles. Feel your hands and fingers mold to her leg. Try single-hand sweeps—especially if she prefers to be held. If she likes it, slide back to the top and start all over!

4   When the massage is over, say, "All done!" and finish off with one final sweep.

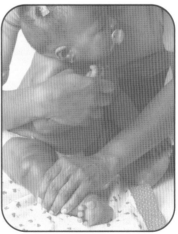

swirl & slide

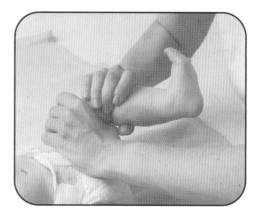

1 Relax and do CLASS.

2 Wrap your hands and fingers in a C shape that molds to the shape of his leg. This is the same placement as Slide & Glide; the difference here is the movement.

3 Swirl your hands so that your elbows move like you were doing a chicken dance while you slide your hands together and away, together and away, down his leg from the upper thigh all the way to the ankle. When your hands slide together, your elbows are up and out (Fig. A). Swirl and slide your hands and fingers away from each other, and let your elbows drop down and in by your sides (Fig. B). If he likes it, slide back to the top of the leg and start all over! You can do this with one hand or two.

4 When the massage is over, say, "All done!" and finish off with one final sweep.

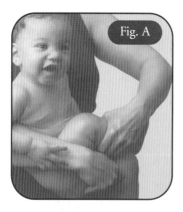

Fig. A

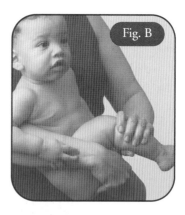

Fig. B

feet and toes

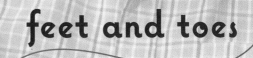

strokes: Sole Slide, Toe Hugs
song suggestion: "B-i-n-g-o"

Feet are fun! Massage can help your baby's feet be less ticklish over time as baby grows familiar with gentle yet firm touch. He's also learning, "I have feet! They're connected to my legs!" This is great body awareness that helps prep him for walking.

sole slide

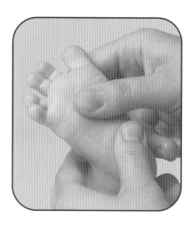

1   Relax and do CLASS.

2   Hold baby's foot at the ankle, with your thumbs at the sole of his foot.

3   Glide your thumb or thumbs across the sole of your baby's foot, heel to toes, in a water-wheel motion.

4   After a few Sole Slides, when you get to the toes, tell a story. As you stroke each toe, name it after a vegetable—a different veggie for each toe. End with toe kisses as you "eat" your vegetable stew! If he likes it, give it another Slide and try a fruit salad!

5   When the massage is over, say, "All done!" and finish off with one final sweep.

touching tip If your prince (or princess) of the castle prefers another position that frees up only one of your thumbs, no problem: just glide a single thumb in the same motion from heel to toes. It's that simple!

toe hugs

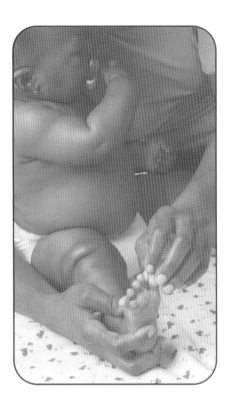

1 Relax and do CLASS.

2 Using your thumb and index finger, hug each of your baby's toes one by one. It doesn't matter if you start with a big toe or a pinky toe.

3 Slide your fingers up, down, and around each toe. Do this until you have hugged all his toes . . . and kisses are nice too! Remember veggies and fruits for yummy stews and salads!

4 When the massage is over, say, "All done!" and finish off with one final sweep.

touching tip Make sure you are not pulling or twisting the toe.

belly

stroke: Belly Walk
song suggestion: "Skidamarink"

Massaging the stomach is a great way to stimulate digestion, get gas and poop moving, and provide relief to your little one. If your baby has just eaten, wait thirty minutes to an hour before beginning a belly massage. For a Tummy-Trouble massage, see page 57.

belly walk

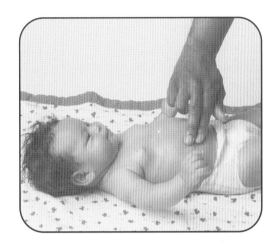

1   Relax and do CLASS.

2   Staying under her rib cage and above her belly button, use the pads of your index and middle fingers from one hand to "moonwalk" across your baby's belly from 10:00-ish to 2:00-ish.

3   Each "step" should be gentle yet firm and slow enough that each finger molds to the baby's body; otherwise, it can tickle. You may feel gas bubbles beneath your fingers!

4   When the massage is over, say, "All done!" and finish off with one final sweep.

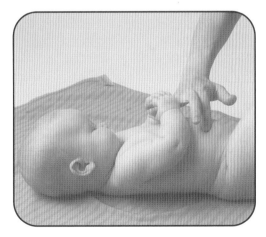

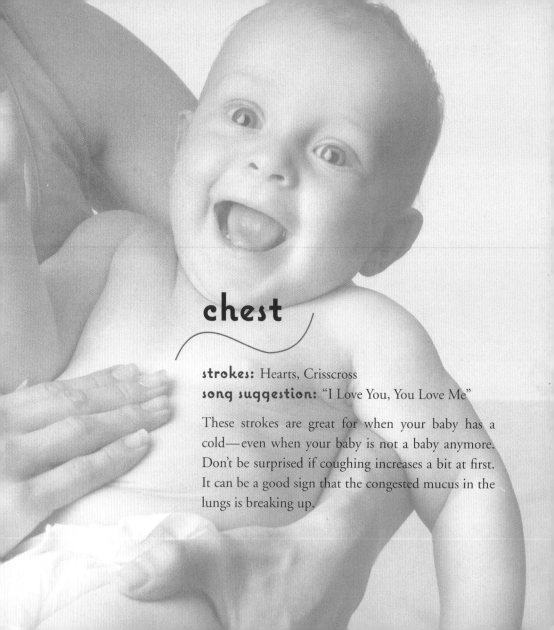

chest

strokes: Hearts, Crisscross

song suggestion: "I Love You, You Love Me"

These strokes are great for when your baby has a cold—even when your baby is not a baby anymore. Don't be surprised if coughing increases a bit at first. It can be a good sign that the congested mucus in the lungs is breaking up.

hearts

1 Relax and do CLASS.

2 Draw a heart:

a Begin with both hands flat in the middle of your baby's chest, just above the bottom end of the rib cage. This is the tip of the heart. Feel your hands mold to your baby's chest.

b In a continual motion, glide your hands together and up the middle of his chest.

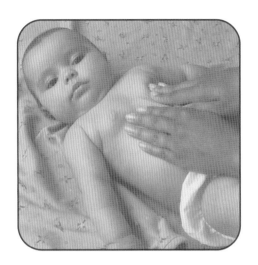

touching tip Do as much as you can without forcing your baby's arms open. If she does not want to open her arms, try this massage another time.

c At the top of his chest, your hands move away from each other, forming the rounded tops of the heart. Glide your hands down and finish drawing the heart shape with your hands meeting together where they started.

3 When the massage is over, say, "All done!" and finish off with one final sweep.

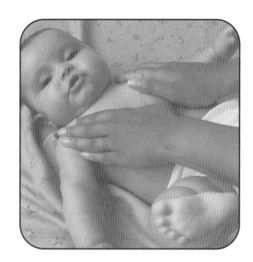

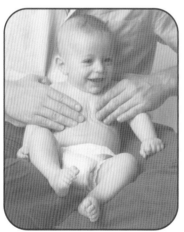

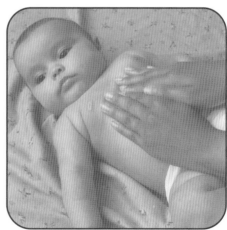

touching tip Does baby want to sit up or be held and look around? No problem!

crisscross

1   Relax and do CLASS.

2   Place your hands flat on either side of the lower half of your baby's chest. Feel your hands mold to his body.

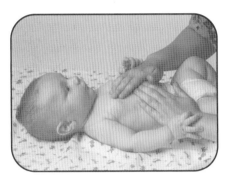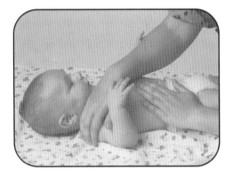

3   Alternate, one hand at a time, in a diagonal stroke up the chest to the opposite shoulder and back down. Crisscross, crisscross. Feel your fingers reach the opposite shoulder; let your fingers curl and give the shoulder a hug. Crisscross, crisscross.

4   When the massage is over, say, "All done!" and finish off with one final sweep.

> **touching tip** To do this one-handed, draw one diagonal crisscross line at a time. Draw it a few times and then switch to the other diagonal line across your baby's chest. This is a good back stroke too—hold your baby in the burping position and you're set!

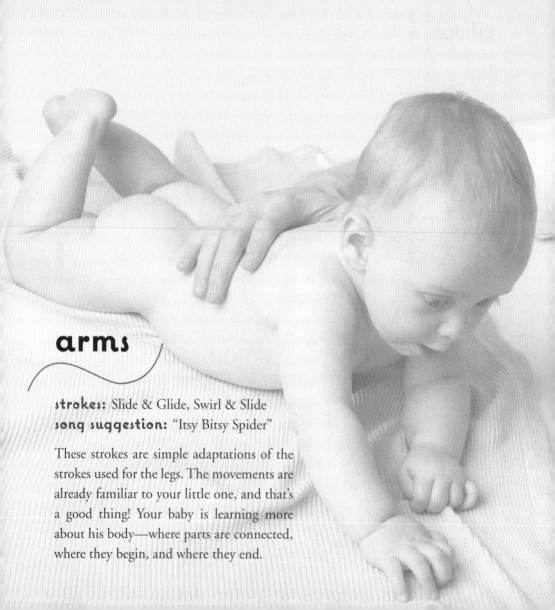

arms

strokes: Slide & Glide, Swirl & Slide
song suggestion: "Itsy Bitsy Spider"

These strokes are simple adaptations of the strokes used for the legs. The movements are already familiar to your little one, and that's a good thing! Your baby is learning more about his body—where parts are connected, where they begin, and where they end.

slide & glide

1   Relax and do CLASS.

2   Wrap your hands around the upper arm, so your fingers make a C shape. Mold your fingers around her arm so there is gentle yet firm contact.

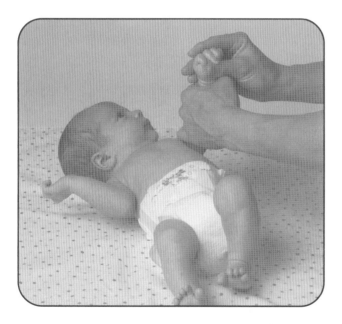

3   Stroke down to the wrist in alternating hand-over-hand motions.

4   When the massage is over, say, "All done!" and finish off with one final sweep.

swirl & slide

1 Relax and do CLASS.

2 With both hands in a C shape, hold your baby's upper arm, one hand on top of the other. Fingers are on top and thumbs are underneath. Glide your hands and fingers together, swirling together and away in alternating glides around his arm as you stroke down to the wrist. Your elbows will move like you were doing a chicken dance. Slide hands and fingers together, and elbows swing up and out. Slide hands and fingers away from each other, and elbows drop down and in by your sides.

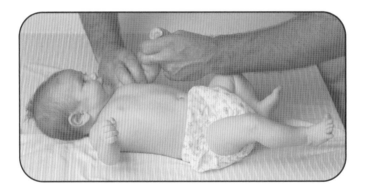

3 When the massage is over, say, "All done!" and finish off with one final sweep.

touching tip If your baby prefers to sit or be held, you can do this single-handed with no problem. Just rotate the Swirl, one-handed, and Glide from the upper arm to the wrist. You're still doing it right!

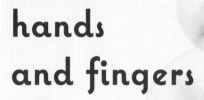

hands and fingers

strokes: Blooming Bud, Finger Hugs
song suggestion: "Five Little Monkeys Jumping on a Bed"

Hands are very hard-working parts of the body—even for a baby—so a hand massage is always welcome. Another wonderful thing about massaging the hands is that you can do it anywhere—while sitting, standing, or even singing and dancing!

blooming bud

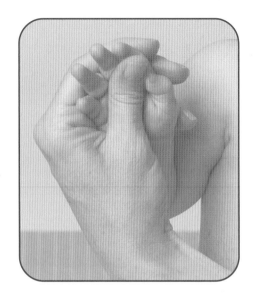

1 Relax and do CLASS.

2 Let the back of baby's hand rest in your palm. Using your thumbs and without forcing your baby to open her hand, stroke through as much of her palm as you can. Stroke from the heel of the palm to the top of the fingers and watch them open— as if a flower bud were opening.

3 When the massage is over, say, "All done!" and finish off with one final sweep.

touching tip Never force the hand open. To encourage your baby to open her hand, try tapping or stroking across the back of her hand. If she still doesn't want to relax her grip, wait for another time.

finger hugs

touching tip This stroke is similar to the toe hug, and again it doesn't matter if you hug thumb-to-pinky or in the opposite direction; the important thing here is that she feels you stroke each of her fingers.

1 Relax and do CLASS.

2 Using the pads of your thumb and index fingers, hug the base of one of your baby's fingers.

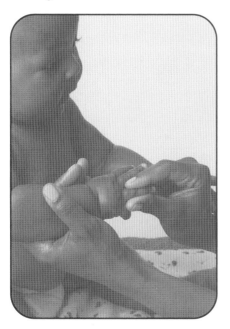

3 With gentle yet firm contact, glide up to the end of her finger, and then around the finger to the next one. Name each finger with a favorite fruit as you massage it. End with finger kisses as you "eat" your fruit salad!

4 When the massage is over, say, "All done!" and finish off with one final sweep.

touching tip Do not pull or twist the finger.

face

stroke: Forehead Fan, Jaw Circles

song suggestion: "Twinkle, Twinkle Little Star"

Just as it is for most grown ups, the face is a very personal space for your baby. It is extra important to do the CLASS routine here to let baby know what's coming. You do not need oil for a face massage, however. If you have some oil on your hands, that's okay; just don't add any more. Even though you're not adding any oil, do the "swish" movement, so the routine stays the same.

forehead fan

1   Relax and do CLASS.

2   Using the pads of your thumbs or index fingers, simultaneously stroke the forehead over each eyebrow. Start at the center of her forehead and follow the brow line out to the sides of her forehead. Tell her, "What beautiful eyes you have!"

3   As usual, if this stroke needs to be performed one-handed, no problem: just do one side at a time!

4   When the massage is over, say, "All done!" and finish off with one final sweep.

> **touching tip** Keep your hands above baby's eyes and do not cover the eyes.

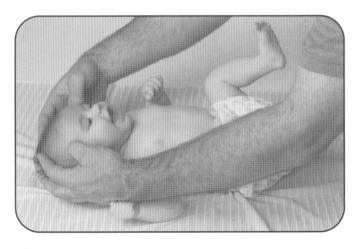

jaw circles

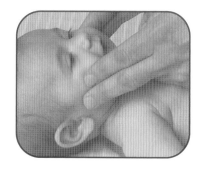

touching tip These feel very good on tiny jaw muscles that are getting a workout from sucking, teething, gnawing, chewing, cooing, and crying!

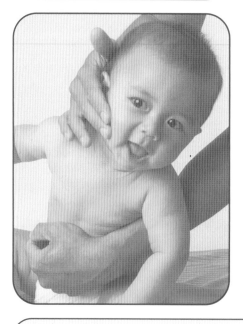

1   Relax and do CLASS.

2   Facing baby, place the pads of your index, middle, and maybe even your ring fingers on your baby's cheeks as if you were holding her face to rub noses or plant a kiss on her forehead. You can rest your thumbs lightly on her chin.

3   Stroke in circles, backward or forward. Look at her and ask, "Does that feel good?"

4   When the massage is over, say, "All done!" and finish off with one final sweep.

touching tip Here, too, if you need to hold baby, use one hand and do one cheek at a time.

back

strokes: Back & Forth, Backside Sweep
song suggestion: "Row, Row, Row Your Boat"

The back is a great baby massage spot, since it presents
a nice large space to work with. If your baby can hold
his head up, place him on his belly horizontally in front
of you. If his head is still wobbly, hold him against you
in the burping position so he can rest his head on you.
Even if he is holding his head up, he might enjoy the
safe, secure feeling of snuggling his head into the soft
warmth of your neck.

back & forth

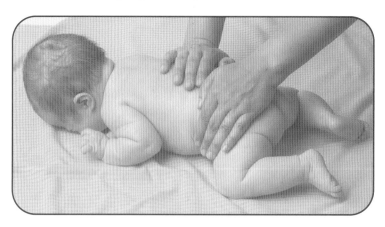

> **touching tip** Never put pressure directly on the spine. Focus on the muscles with a light yet firm touch.

1 Relax and do CLASS.

2 Relax and soften your hands, placing them on his back at his shoulders. Your hands should be placed across his back, fingers pointing across his spine. Let him feel the warmth and security of your hands.

3 Glide one hand forward while the other glides back—back and forth, back and forth—in alternating motions across his back. As you glide across his back, your hands should naturally cup over his spine.

4 You can start at the top of his back and work down to his bottom or start at his bottom and work your way up to the top of his back.

5 When the massage is over, say, "All done!" and finish off with one final sweep.

> **touching tip** If your baby prefers to be held, try stroking with one hand back and forth across his back.

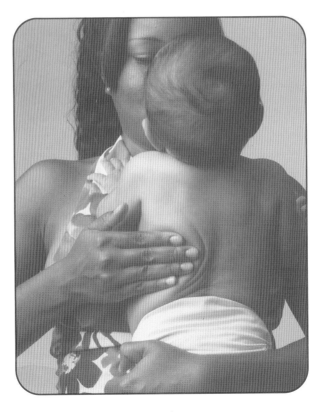

backside sweep

> **touching tip** This is a great body awareness opportunity for your baby to feel his entire back from top to bottom.

1 Relax and do CLASS.

2 Hands relaxed and resting on your baby's back, start at the top of his back and swoop all the way down to his ankles.

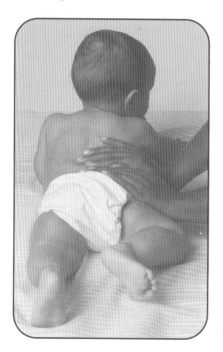
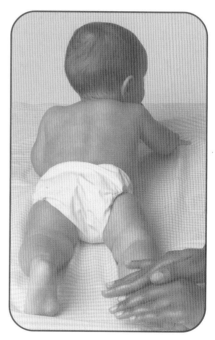

3 If he's belly down and in front of you, use both hands, one on each side of his back. Start at the top of his back and swoop all the way down to his ankles, both sides at one time.

4 If you're holding him, sweep one side at a time all the way down to each ankle.

5 When the massage is over, say, "All done!" and finish off with one final sweep.

touching tip Do *not* put direct pressure on the spine.

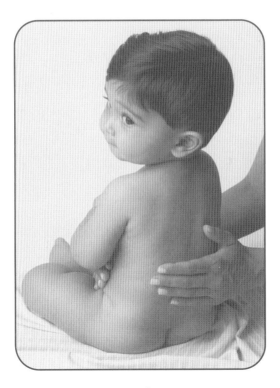

special massages

These massages are intended to offer you ideas on how to create more special time with your baby. They can be a routine that your baby comes to enjoy or they can be spontaneous massages you do whenever you can. Remember: this is baby-focused time that is good for both of you.

morning wakey-wakey massage

song suggestion: The first verse of "Zip-a-Dee-Do-Da"
slide & glide upward: Arms and legs

> **touching tip** The upward movement of these two strokes is invigorating, and it's a great way for you and your baby to start your day in sync.

1 Relax and do CLASS.

2 Mold your hands in a C shape to your baby's arm or leg.

3 For legs, Slide & Glide from the ankle to the top of the leg.

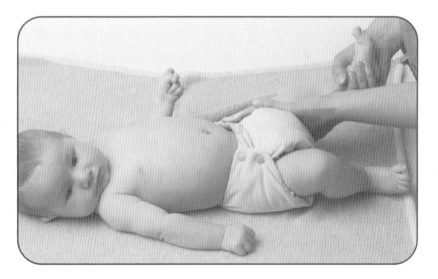

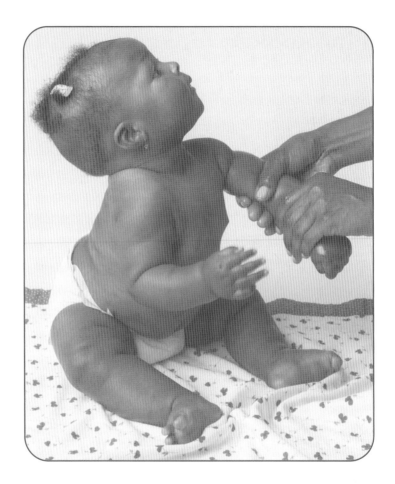

4   For the arms, Slide & Glide from the wrist to the top of the arm.

5   When the massage is over, say, "All done!" and finish off with one final sweep.

bath-time bubble massage

song suggestion: First verse of "You Are My Sunshine"
swirl & slide: Legs
hearts and crisscross: Chest

Bath time can be a perfect time to get in a massage. Your hands are slippery with water and bubbles and you're naturally massaging your baby already! Use your hands, a sponge, or a washcloth. If you feel that massaging baby in the bathtub is too slippery or insecure, do it while you're drying him off. Remember: one-handed strokes are just fine. Do what is comfortable and works best for you. Just be sure he doesn't eat the bubbles, and rinse your baby off well!

1   Relax and do CLASS.

2   Swirl & Slide down your baby's legs from the upper leg to the ankles. First one leg, then the other.

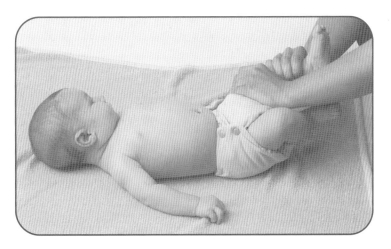

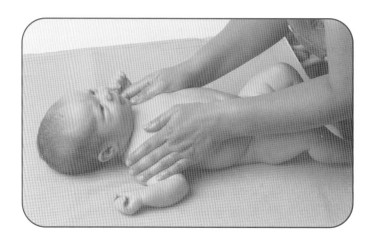

3 Draw Hearts and Crisscrosses on your baby's chest.

4 When the massage is over, say, "All done!" and finish off with one final sweep.

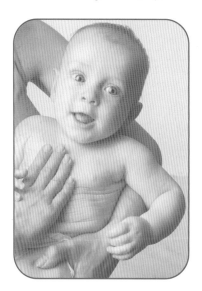

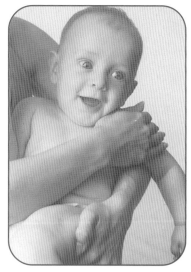

tummy-trouble massage

This massage can be part of your standard routine, but you will want to use it especially when your baby is constipated or gassy, which can make him fussy. This massage is best to do when your baby is not having a colicky episode. Use a soothing tone to tell him that you understand he's uncomfortable and that you are doing your best to help him feel better.

1 Relax and do CLASS.

2 With both palms, make good contact with your baby's belly and imagine a clock. Begin stroking in a clockwise motion—the direction that gas and poop move in—around the belly button and under the rib cage.

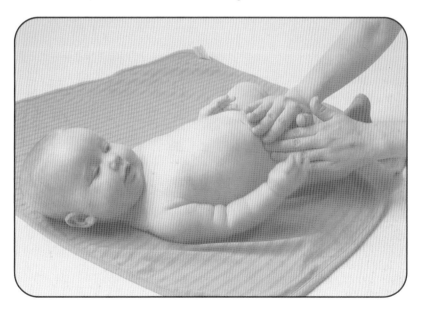

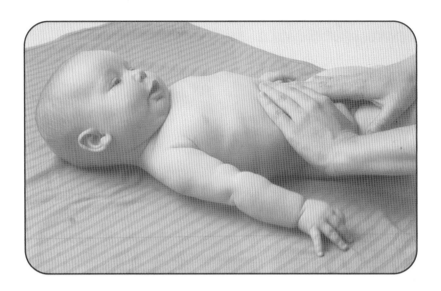

3 Your left hand will keep moving around all the hours on the clock. The right hand follows the left hand, moving from 10:00-ish to 5:00-ish, as if the hands were chasing each other.

4 A one-handed stroke comes in handy when your baby prefers sitting in your lap and seeing the world. Make good contact and stroke clockwise around the belly button and underneath the rib cage.

5 When the massage is over, say, "All done!" and finish off with one final sweep.

touching tip Don't be astonished if you get a surprise delivery in that diaper or on that blanket. In a baby's world, this is good news! Celebrate!

sleepy-time massage

suggestion: This is a great time for your child's favorite bedtime song, rhyme, or story.
slide & glide downward: Arms and legs
backside sweep downward: Back and legs

> **touching tip** When it's time to sleep, stroking slowly downward can help you both relax.

1   Relax and do CLASS.

2   Hands relaxed and molded to your baby's body, Slide & Glide down one arm at a time from her upper arm to her wrist.

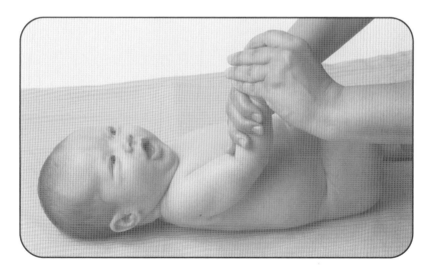

3   Slide & Glide down one leg at a time from her upper thigh to her ankle.

4   If your baby is on her belly or you're holding her, use slow sweeping motions down her back and down each leg to the ankle.

> **touching tip** Watch your baby's cues; as her eyes start to get heavy, you can continue to cuddle or sing softly, but now slow down the strokes even more and end by just holding your hands still. When you are ready to leave, do it slowly and whisper, "All done." She'll be more likely not to notice as she enters a deep sleep.

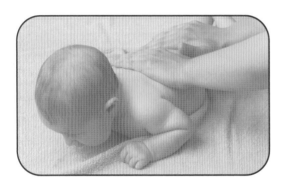

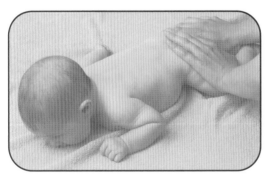

conclusion

Thanks to you, your baby is growing up happy and healthy. Her brain is busily making connections, and she's learning that she owns her body. The immediate benefit is that every time you touch each other, smile at each other, laugh together, and gaze into each other's eyes, your relationship is growing as well. You are sharing experiences and providing a foundation for a strong and healthy lifelong bond.

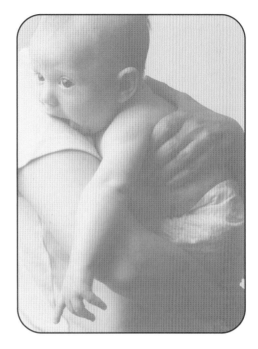

For a more in-depth look into the history and traditions of baby massage, please refer to the work of two people who are the inspirations for this book: Dr. Frederick Leboyer, author of *Loving Hands: The Art of Baby Massage,* and Vimala McClure, author of *Infant Massage: A Handbook for Loving Parents.* In the 1970s, they pioneered the study and practice of baby massage in the West, and McClure founded the first nonprofit organization for baby massage. Their books are considered classics on the subject of baby massage.

meet the models

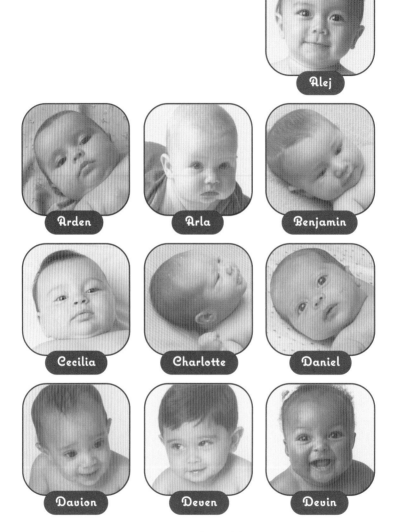

Alej

Arden

Arla

Benjamin

Cecilia

Charlotte

Daniel

Davion

Deven

Devin

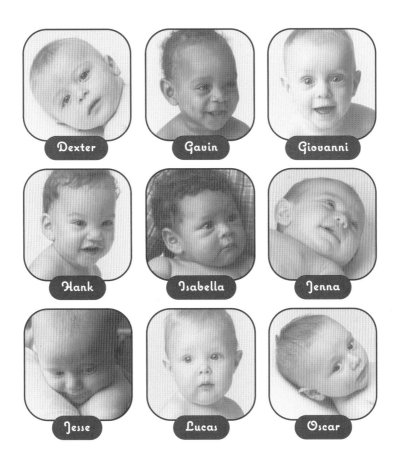

buzz sources

For more research abstracts on the benefits of massage for infants and children, visit the Touch Resource Institute's Web site: www.miami.edu/touch-research/index.html.

1

Ferber, S., et al. 2002. Massage therapy by mothers enhances the adjustment of circadian rhythms to the nocturnal period in full-term infants. *Journal of Developmental & Behavioral Pediatrics* 23, no. 6 (December): 410–15.

Field, T., & M. Hernandez-Reif. 2001. Sleep problems in infants decrease following massage therapy. *Early Child Development and Care* 168: 95–104.

2

Cigales, M., et al. 1997. Massage enhances recovery from habituation in normal infants. *Infant Behavior and Development* 20: 29–34.

3

Field, T. 1998. Effects of massage therapy. *American Psychologist* 53 (12): 1270–81

4

Field, T., et al. 1996. Massage and relaxation therapies' effects on depressed adolescent mothers. *Adolescence* 31: 903–11.

5

Pelaez-Nogueras, M., et al. 1996. Depressed mothers' touching increases infants' positive affect and attention in still-face interactions. *Child Development* 67: 1780–92.

5

Field, T., et al. 1996. Massage therapy for infants of depressed mothers. *Infant Behavior and Development* 19: 109–14.

6

Cullen, C., et al. 2000. Father-infants interactions are enhanced by massage therapy. *Early Child Development and Care* 164: 41–47.

7

Scafidi, F., & T. Field. 1997. Massage therapy improves behavior in neonates born to HIV positive mothers. *Journal of Pediatric Psychology* 21: 889–97.

8

Dieter, J., et al. 2003. Preterm infants gain more weight and sleep less following five days of massage therapy. *Journal of Pediatric Psychology* 28 (6): 403–11.

9

Plaja, F., & M. Alesi. 2004. Pain in newborns and children. *Prof Inferm* 57, no. 3 (July–September): 135–38.

song credits

"Wheels on the Bus"
Author Unknown

"B-i-n-g-o"
Author Unknown

"Skidamarink"
Author Unknown

"I Love You, You Love Me"
Lyrics by Lee Bernstein

"Itsy Bitsy Spider"
Author Unknown

"Five Little Monkeys Jumping on a Bed"
Author Unknown

"Twinkle, Twinkle Little Star"
Author Unknown

"Row, Row, Row Your Boat"
Author Unknown

"You Are My Sunshine"
Written by former Louisiana governor
Jimmie Davis and Charles Mitchell;
copyright 1940 and 1977 by Peer
International Corporation

"Zip-a-Dee-Do-Da"
Music by Allie Wrubel; lyrics by Ray
Gilbert

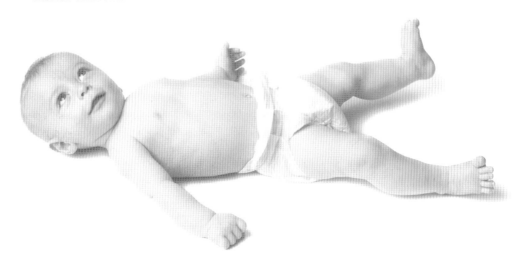

index

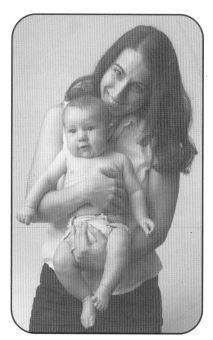

Suzanne P. Reese lives in the desert mountains of San Diego County, California, with her husband and their dog. She is of Armenian and Argentine descent, and her baby massage experiences started when she was, well, a baby! Bubbly massages were routine during bath time with Nanny (Suzanne's maternal grandmother). When Suzanne caught a cold or flu bug, nightly massages by Dad were sure to deliver a better night's sleep. Mom was the best for comforting holds and hugs—and still is. Suzanne is a Certified International Infant Massage Instructor-trainer and parent educator. Her academic background includes an undergraduate degree in child development and national certification in therapeutic massage and bodywork. She is a member of the International Association of Infant Massage (IAIM). Suzanne travels across the United States and around the globe sharing the tradition, science, and fun of baby massage. She leads intensive training workshops and makes presentations at international conferences. Suzanne is committed to the evolution of healthy parent-infant bonding and infant development through nurturing and compassionate touch. She extends an age-old approach to the care of infants and children that can be adapted to the fast pace of our daily modern lives. To learn more about Suzanne or to contact her, please visit www.compassionatechild.com.